Introduction

EMERGENCY SURVIVAL
a pocket guide

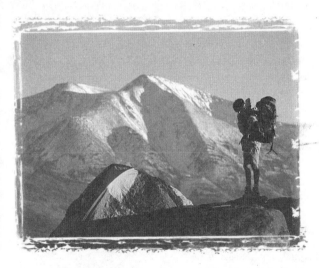

Quick Information for Outdoor Safety

Christopher Van Tilburg, M.D.

THE MOUNTAINEERS BOOKS

Published by
The Mountaineers Books
1001 SW Klickitat Way, Suite 201
Seattle, WA 98134

© 2001 by The Mountaineers Books

First printing 2001, second printing 2004, third printing 2006,
fourth printing 2007, fifth printing 2008, sixth printing 2009,
seventh printing 2011

Distributed in the United Kingdom by Cordee, www.cordee.co.uk

Manufactured in the United States of America

Project Editor: Julie Van Pelt
Copy Editor: Chris DeVito
Cover and Book Design: Kristy Welch and Mayumi Thompson
Layout: Mayumi Thompson
Illustrator: Scott Gaudette

ISBN: 978-0-89886-768-8

+ Introduction +

Wilderness survival is one skill that we hope to never need. However, when survival is necessary for whatever reason—accident, illness, losing one's way, or inclement weather—it always comes at a time that is unexpected. So above all, always be ready for survival situations, however large or small.

This booklet has limitations, like all instruction texts. Written in outline form, it serves as a reminder of skills learned previously and practiced regularly. It will jog your memory and help formulate decisions based on your preexisting knowledge of survival.

This booklet does not explain recommended skills and procedures in detail, but rather highlights the main points. It does not cover every situation or possible scenario but tries to include the most common skills that may be necessary and summarizes the steps briefly. It should be preceded by practical survival and first-aid training, routine practice of the skills, and regular updates. Without them, this book is not much use.

Prevention is the cornerstone of safety. There is no substitute for using proper judgment, employing caution, being prepared, and using your brain. No matter what the activity, climate, or area, wilderness and outdoor adventures always have some level of risk involved. You should accept this risk.

No text can realistically discuss all survival issues, nor can it compensate for the limitations of readers. There is no substitute for certified survival instruction, routine practice of survival techniques, experience, and regular updates of new information. The survival skills outlined here are meant as brief reminders of information learned from other sources such as full-length survival books and survival courses. This book has been researched using material thought to be the most accurate and up to date. However, this is not guaranteed. Readers should understand that omissions, typographical errors, and other mistakes are possible. Readers should take all responsibility for wilderness survival situations.

✦ Preparation ✦

Preparation is the key to any survival situation. Before you go, follow some basic principals:

1. Mental preparation is crucial. Survival experts, as well as wilderness adventurers in life-or-death situations, continue to reinforce that mental outlook is vital for survival situations. The will to survive, perseverance, and hope are the mainstays of the survival mentality. Avoid and be ready to deal with anxiety, fear, and guilt.

2. Physical preparation is equally important. You should be in good physical condition. This means regular workouts for strength, endurance, and cardiovascular conditioning. Always stay within your skill level and physical limits.

3. Formal instruction in wilderness travel and survival is mandatory. Regular practice and routine updates in information are important to keep skills fresh, especially those that are not used on a regular basis. Read and reread survival books.

4. Take cardiopulmonary resuscitation (CPR) and first-aid courses and study wilderness first-aid books.

5. Gather equipment and check, repair, and replace parts if needed. Change batteries in electronics. Replace first-aid and survival kit components that are outdated or were used on a previous trip.

6. Choose your partners wisely: They should have skills and mental and physical conditioning similar to yours. Remember, in a survival situation, you may be relying on them.

7. Plan your route and leave it with someone. Allow for changes in plan due to route or weather conditions.

8. Continually reevaluate road, trail, and weather conditions and forecasts. Check with rangers for updates on conditions. Confirm camping and trail permits.
9. Be prepared to abandon the trip if weather, trail, or other conditions are not safe.

When afield, additional measures should be followed both to prevent and maximally prepare yourself for a survival situation.
1. Constantly evaluate trail, route, and weather conditions.
2. Always stay within the limits of your and your partners' skill and equipment. Use good judgment and don't take unnecessary risks.
3. Always stay well hydrated and well nourished.
4. Make sure everyone is well rested; take regular breaks.
5. Make sure your equipment is working and your clothing is dry.
6. Keep your group in good spirits.
7. For safety, never be afraid to alter your route, cut your trip short, or turn back.

Essentials

There are essential items one should never be without, ever. These basic emergency items should be with you at all times, even on short trips. The essentials in Table 1 make up the baseline list, but keep in mind that this list should be modified and/or expanded depending on the nature of the trip being planned. Snow travel might require an avalanche beacon that would be irrelevant on a desert trip. The extra food, water, and clothing should be above and beyond what you expect to use for your trip. Sometimes this is an extra water bottle, an energy bar, a windbreaker, and minimal survival and first-aid kits. Other times this may be an entire extra day's worth of food and water and enough clothing to spend an unexpected night out. It is best to always have enough supplies to spend at least one unexpected night in the wilderness.

Table 1: Essentials

First-aid kit
Survival kit
GPS and GPS-compatible map, compass, altimeter
Sunglasses
Sunscreen, lip balm
Flashlight or headlamp, extra batteries
Extra food and water
Extra clothing
Bivouac sack or tarp
Radio or cell phone

Survival Kit

Numerous survival and emergency kits are available from commercial companies and outfitters. Buy one that suits your needs, or you can assemble your own. In general, the contents of your kit depend on how long you will be out in the field, your survival skills, the number of people in your party, how far from help you will be, and the type of activity you are pursuing. Special equipment is required for travel in the mountains, in water, in desert, or in tropical jungle. If involved in sports such as paddling, biking, skiing, snowboarding, or climbing, carry repair equipment for those activities. This may include repairs for ski/snowboard bindings, leaks in rafts, broken bike derailer or chain, flat tires, and other such mishaps.

A minimal survival kit (Table 2) can be used for short trips in mild weather, such as a half-day hike in summer. Keep in mind, this is the bare minimum. It is designed to fit in a coat pocket, fanny pack, or day pack.

Table 2: Minimal Survival Kit

Bandages, small
First-aid or duct tape
Firestarter
Matches, lighter, flint
GPS and GPS-compatible map, compass, altimeter
Radio or cell phone
Safety pin
Sunscreen, small tube
Pocket tool (with pliers, wire cutter, screwdrivers,
    tweezers, scissors, awl, knife)
Water purification tablets
Whistle

An expanded survival kit (Table 3) with more items is necessary for longer trips, such as long day hikes, or overnight backpacking. You will also need more than the minimal survival kit for rigorous activity, such as climbing, mountaineering, or other adventure sports.

Table 3: Expanded Survival Kit

Batteries, two AA or other
Cable ties, two, 7.5-inch plastic
Chemical hand/foot warmers, two
Cord, 10 feet × 4 mm Perlon
Duct tape, 2 inches × 5 feet
Firestarter
Insect repellent

Match container, waterproof
Matches (windproof, waterproof), lighter, flint
Needle (heavy gauge) and nylon thread
Pen and paper
Pocket tool (with pliers, wire cutter, screwdrivers,
    tweezers, scissors, awl, knife)
Repair items, activity specific
Safety pins
Signal mirror
Sunscreen
Water purification tablets
Wire
Whistle

A vehicle survival kit is designed to assist you if your vehicle breaks down, gets stuck, or otherwise leaves you stranded (Table 4).

Table 4: Vehicle Survival Kit
Fire extinguisher
Flares
Food and water
Gas, extra
Jack and tire iron
Jumper cables
Light, battery powered
Motor oil, extra
Repair tools
Sand plate (jack stand for sand, snow, mud)
Shovel
Spare tire

Tire pump
Tow chain or strap

First-Aid Kit

First-aid kits are highly variable. Like survival kits, first-aid materials depend on how long you will be out in the field, your first-aid skills, the number of people in your party, how far from help you will be, and the type of activity you are pursuing. Remember that special items may be required for travel at high elevation, in water, in the tropics, or in the desert. Also, if you don't know how to use the equipment, it is useless. Some items can be replaced by improvisation, such as splint or bandage material.

A basic first-aid kit for general travel in mild climates works for basic backpacking, hiking, or biking (Table 5). It generally covers wound care. This is a bare minimum for a short hike or bike, or a day skiing in a resort. It is small enough to fit in a fanny pack, parka pocket, camera bag, or the like. If it is too bulky, you may not want to carry it for a short trip. Keep in mind that this leaves out several items you may deem essential, such as moleskin. Note: Some items in your first-aid kit may already be part of the essentials or survival kit, such as sunscreen and water purification tablets.

Table 5: Basic First-Aid Kit

Antiseptic wipe
Bandages, several sizes
Bio-occlusive dressing
Benzoin crush tube
Butterfly bandages, large
First-aid tape
Gauze, 4×4 inch, 2×2 inch

Gauze roll or triangle bandage
Gloves and CPR microshield
Sunscreen

A more comprehensive first-aid kit should be carried for day hikes, on longer trips, on overnight trips, in a car, and whenever you are doing higher-risk activities such as mountaineering, climbing, mountain biking, or paddling (Table 6). This is a general kit that you need to customize for your trip, especially if you are involved in water sports or high-altitude mountaineering.

Table 6: Expanded First-Aid Kit

Antibacterial cleanser
Antibacterial ointment
Anti-inflammatory medication (ibuprofen)
Antihistamine (diphenhydramine)
Adhesive bandages
Benzoin
Bio-occlusive dressing
Butterfly bandages
First-aid book
First-aid tape
Gauze, 4 × 4 inch, 2 × 2 inch
Gloves and CPR microshield
Hydrocortisone cream
Moleskin
Multiuse tool (tweezers, knife, scissors)
Needle
Nonadherent dressing
Oral rehydration powder

Pen, paper, accident report form
Roll (2 inch) or triangle bandage
Safety pins
Splint, malleable
Sunscreen
Syringe
Thermometer
Water purification tablets

✦ Surviving in the Wilderness ✦

General Survival Procedures

Survival procedures depend on the situation, and no one algorithm can fully address all issues. However, some general principals should always be followed.

When an accident or situation occurs, quickly assess the situation and make an initial plan. Some things require quick thinking and immediate action; life-threatening situations must be dealt with. This may include rendering first aid, initiating avalanche search, or performing water rescue. Above all, safety of the group and uninjured or unaffected partners is paramount; don't risk additional injury. The situation should be continually reassessed because it will probably be in a constant state of change.

Once immediate situations are addressed, you should make a thorough assessment of the scene. Important assessment tools include the following: gather all your partners; assess equipment and skills available; evaluate your supplies of food, water, and clothing; and evaluate the mental and physical health of everyone in your group. Above all, stay calm and avoid panic, anxiety, fear, and guilt.

Sometimes a leader is established for larger groups. This is often the person with the most survival, outdoor, or first-aid experience. However, in tight-knit groups, everyone may act as a leader, and decisions may be mutual.

Establish a priority right away. Sometimes tasks should be completed in a stepwise fashion; sometimes they are completed simultaneously. For example, one person may render first aid to an injured person while a second procures water and a third begins finding shelter.

For establishing priorities, no one list or set of guidelines can address all situations; a rough listing of priority follows.

1. Immediate priority should be given to evaluating and treating injuries; procuring water if supply is low; making sure everyone has adequate warm, dry clothing; and creating an evacuation plan if necessary.
2. High-priority tasks include finding your way if lost; following through with an evacuation plan; finding and building shelter; preparing for travel; and using radios or cell phones, if available.
3. Lower-priority tasks (for example, if you are in a multi-day survival situation) include building a fire; signaling rescuers, when appropriate; and procuring food.

Evacuation Plan
When a survival situation occurs, you will usually need to make an initial plan to deal with life-threatening emergencies, followed by a more detailed plan for evacuation. Usually this is one of three situations: continuing with the trip, evacuating, or staying put and getting help. Special concerns outlined later pertain to an injury to a member of your group.

Occasionally, you can continue your trip. For example, if your chief problem is low water, you may be able to employ skills to procure water, and then continue with your trip. A small cut may need only basic first aid. Remember, however, that even a seemingly minor situation can turn disastrous. So if you choose to continue with your trip, make sure this is a wise and prudent decision.

For most survival situations, you will need to abort the trip. Initially, you should decide whether you should stay put or evacuate. There are several components to the decision. First, consider the type of situation. For example, a major life-threatening injury may require the injured person to stay put while others go for help. Likewise, if you are caught in foul weather and become lost, it may be better to stay in one place until the weather subsides. On the other hand, basic problems such as running out of food or water may require you to abandon your trip and go home.

Other factors that should be considered when making a decision include time and distance needed for evacuation, survival skills of group members, available equipment and clothing, quantities of food and water, suitable bivouac sites, available materials for shelter, current weather conditions and forecast, time left until nightfall, injuries sustained by group members, condition of the route and the feasibility of reversing it, and other factors.

Above all, survival situations are highly variable, and you must take all possibilities into account. Similarly, survival situations usually change at some point, so reevaluate the situation on a regular basis. Try to stick to your plan, but don't be so strict that you are unwilling to alter your evacuation plan for safety.

If you decide to abort the trip, get out quickly but safely. Don't take unnecessary risks. Don't risk injury. If necessary, you may need to bivouac for the night and then evacuate the next day. Be wary of shortcuts; you can get lost easier if you are off route, and off-trail travel may be difficult.

If you decide to stay put, begin procuring water and building a shelter. If needed, gather firewood before dark. Organize your gear. Consider trying to initiate a rescue with a cell phone or radio. Begin survival prioritizing as outlined previously.

Evacuating an injured or ill person is more complicated. For minor injures, if the injured person can walk, this is a fast and safe method for evacuation. If the injured person cannot walk, you may need to carry him or her out. For severe injuries in which moving the person is difficult or contraindicated, you may need to send one person for help and leave extra food, water, clothing, sleeping equipment, and a cooking set with the injured person. Remember, with a head or spine injury, only trained personnel should move the injured person. With large groups, you can have some people go for help while others stay in a bivouac.

Regarding rescue that requires technical equipment and skill, it is best not to attempt this if you have neither skills nor equipment. This may include crevasse, high-angle rock, and swift-water rescues. It is easy to cause additional injury, so these situations are best left for rescuers.

Regarding rescue with helicopters, it is worth noting a few points. A landing zone should be at least 100 by 300 feet and marked with bright clothing or packs. Secure equipment before the helicopter approaches. If the helicopter lowers gear, let it touch the ground first to dissipate static electricity. Protect yourself and others from flying debris. Watch the top rotor and the rear rotor; both can be difficult to see. Approach the cabin from the front, bending low to the ground, only when signaled to do so by pilot. For communicating with air rescue teams and helicopter pilots, see Signaling below.

Signaling

If you have decided to wait for rescue, as described above, several things can increase your chance of being seen. Keep in mind that rescue is often not initiated until you are reported missing. This may be several days. If you are injured and part of your group went for help, stay put if your location is known by your partner. This will speed rescue. If you are lost, stay put; traveling blindly may prolong rescue.

1. Spread out your tarp and bright-colored clothing.
2. Use your whistle if rescuers are nearby.
3. Waving may help if aircraft are searching. Try waving bright-colored clothing or your tarp.
4. A signal mirror can be used to attract searchers in aircraft or on the ground with line of site. Use the hole in the middle to direct the sun's reflection to the searchers.
5. Smoke from fire may help. Consider burning downed green branches or leaves to increase smoke.
6. On snow or sand, use downed wood, dirt, or clothing to make a large X in a clearing.
7. A cell phone or radio may be used if available. Remember that it may not work due to unavailability of signal, dead batteries, extreme cold, or damage.
8. Ground-to-air signaling patterns may be helpful. Construct large letters by using materials at hand, as depicted in Table 7. On snow use downed logs or dirt to provide contrast.

9. If you must leave the location where your partners left you or where you may be looked for, mark your trail and direction of travel. Use sticks, rocks, or dirt pointing in your direction of travel.
10. Helicopter hand signals are useful for communicating with a rescue pilot, as described in Table 8. For details on a landing zone and helicopter safety, see Evacuation Plan.

Table 7: Ground-to-air Signals

Signal	Meaning	Signal	Meaning
I	Require doctor, serious injury	L⌐	Aircraft seriously damaged
II	Require medical supplies	△	Probably safe to land here
X	Unable to proceed	L	Require fuel
F	Require food and water	LL	All well
□	Require map and compass	N	No
I (dotted)	Require radio	Y	Yes
K	Indicate direction to proceed	⌐L⌐	Not understood
↗	Am proceeding in this direction		

Table 8: Helicopter Hand Signals

Signal	Meaning
Wave arms side to side across body and overhead	Do not land
Stand with back to wind, arms pointed to landing area	Land here, back to wind
Hold out arms with fists closed	Hold your hover
Hold arms out at 45 degrees to ground, with thumbs down	Hold on ground
Move hand across neck	Shut off engine

Low-Impact Survival

Survival situations can be tense and stressful. However, you should still follow low-impact wilderness travel and camping whenever possible.

1. Follow the time-tested mantras: "Take nothing but pictures, leave nothing but footprints, kill nothing but time," and "Pack it in, pack it out."
2. Stay within your skill level. If you are on a route too difficult for your skills, often you trample or destroy fragile environments.
3. Travel in smaller groups.
4. Choose a season and weather consistent with good route conditions. Muddy or dry trails can be particularly damaged.
5. Only drive on designated roads.
6. Ride bikes only on roads or on trails designated for bikes.

7. Take kayaks, rafts, and boats only on waterways where they are allowed.

8. When hiking, stay on trails; avoid taking shortcuts or hiking around mudholes or switchbacks.

9. Don't trample plants, moss, or fragile macrobiotic soil.

10. Avoid animals and their dens. View them from a distance.

11. Manage your waste correctly, as discussed under Human Waste.

12. When bivouacking, set up your tent or tarp in an area that is protected as much as possible. Avoid moving large rocks or logs. If constructing an emergency shelter, use only downed sticks, logs, and tree bows for shelter or padding.

13. For fires, use downed wood. Build the fire in a dry stream bed or area clear of vegetation. Remove your fire ring or fire pit and scatter wet, cold ashes.

Procuring Water

Water is of primary importance in a survival situation. Like shelter, it is paramount to survival. In the wilderness, with strenuous activity, you need about a gallon of water daily. You may need more with prolonged vigorous activity or in high-altitude or very hot climates. Plan well and you'll have an ample supply.

Water can be procured from streams, springs, and lakes. If you have no surface water, you may be able to find water in dry riverbeds by digging below the cutbanks. Other places to dig for water include near plants and below cliffs.

In the mountains, snow is often the only source of water. You will need a stove to melt snow. Eating snow can cause you to lose body heat.

In the deserts, a solar still may need to be constructed (fig. 1). Dig a hole and place a cup in the center. Place brackish water, urine, vegetation, and other sources in the hole, but not in the cup. Place a clear plastic sheet over the hole and weight it with a small rock so that the sheet drops into the center of the cup. As the water evaporates from the hole, it condenses on the underside of the sheet and then drips into the cup. After several hours there may be some drinkable water. Running a straw from the cup to the topsheet allows you to drink water from the cup without tearing down the still.

There are many variations of solar stills that can be used with vegetation. Wrap a bag around tree or brush foliage with a rock weighted in the bottom to collect water.

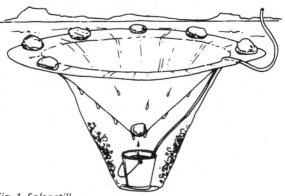

Fig. 1. Solar still

Unless water is acquired by boiling snow, a solar still, or a spring, it should be treated for germs. There are three main methods: chemical, boiling, and mechanical.

Chemical treatment purifies water. Usually iodine tablets are used. They work quickly, but the taste is poor and sometimes too much of this chemical may be harmful. Another option is chlorine bleach or povidone-iodine first-aid cleanser: a few drops in a liter of water will purify it in a half hour.

Boiling works well if you are already melting snow. However, you need to carry a lot of fuel to boil drinking water, and this gets cumbersome and heavy.

There are numerous mechanical devices that either filter or purify water. A filter eliminates many germs but not harmful viruses. A purifier is a filter that is impregnated with a chemical to fully purify water. These are easy and quick to use but add a little weight to your gear.

Lost

Losing your way in the wilderness can be frightening. Sometimes you can check your map and reorient yourself quickly. Other times it may just be a short backtrack to find your trail. Once in a while, however, people become totally lost in the backcountry. If you do, follow a stepwise method:

1. Keep your cool and don't panic.
2. Take a quick break for food and water if needed.
3. Use your map, compass, altimeter, and global positioning system (if available) to locate your position and then plot your route.
4. If poor weather blocks your view of terrain, proceed with extreme caution. You don't want to walk off a cliff or into water.

5. If you can easily find your trail, retracing your steps may be the simplest procedure.

6. If nearby, hike to a ridge or vista that may help you get a view of the trail. Avoid blindly hiking because you may get further from your trail.

7. If late in the day, make a bivouac with your camping gear, or improvise a shelter if needed. Procure water and gather firewood if needed before dark.

8. Consider using a cell phone or radio for help, but remember that self-reliance is of utmost importance. Phones and radios often don't work in the wilderness. Even then, search is limited due to weather, personnel, and other factors.

Navigation

Map, compass, and altimeter navigation is the primary method for wilderness routefinding. Learn to use them and practice often. The compass (fig. 2) has two primary functions: identifying your position on a map and finding your way in the wilderness.

There is an important difference between magnetic north, where the compass points, and true north, where north on a map points. The difference between the two is called declination and must be adjusted for with each compass reading. If possible, use a compass with a built-in declination correction.

You should carry and know how to read a topographic map. The standard for routefinding is the United States Geologic Survey 7.5-minute series (1:24,000 scale).

A brief synopsis of map and compass navigation follows.

Locating Your Position

1. Identify a landmark in the field.

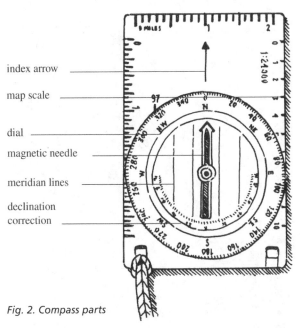

index arrow

map scale

dial

magnetic needle

meridian lines

declination
correction

Fig. 2. Compass parts

2. Locate the corresponding landmark on the topographic map.
3. Take a field bearing by aiming the compass arrow at the landmark in the field and turning the dial so that north on the dial lines up with the needle pointing to magnetic north
4. Read the bearing at the arrow.
5. Convert your field bearing to a map bearing by adding or subtracting the number of degrees of declination. The topographic map should list the declination correction; it differs depending on your location. Follow directions on

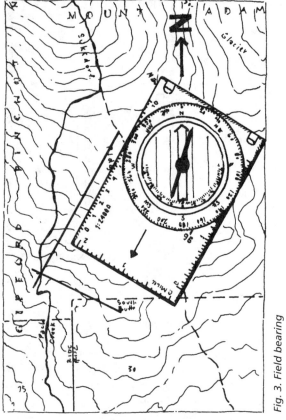

Fig. 3. Field bearing

your compass instructions for conversion. If you have a basic
compass you can manually adjust this. For a west declination,
turn the dial clockwise the correct number of degrees. For

an east declination, turn the dial counterclockwise.

6. Put the compass on the map, align the compass with the landmark on the map, and turn the entire compass so that north on the dial is aligned with north on the map. Scribe a line. Your position is along this bearing (fig. 3).

7. Repeat the steps with a second landmark. Your position is marked at the point where the two lines intersect.

Finding a Route

1. Locate your position as described above.

2. Acquire a map bearing by placing the compass edge on your position and on the location toward which you are headed, and then turn the dial so north is aligned with north on the map (fig. 4).

3. Read the bearing at the arrow.

4. Convert your map bearing to a field bearing by adding or subtracting the degrees of declination. The topographic map should list the declination correction; it differs depending on your location. Follow the directions on your compass instructions for conversion. If you have a basic compass, manually adjust this. For a west declination, turn the dial counterclockwise the correct number of degrees. For an east declination, turn the dial clockwise.

5. While holding the compass level, turn the entire unit so the needle and dial on the compass point to magnetic north. The arrow points to your direction of travel.

Altimeter

An altimeter is very useful when identifying your position or finding your way. The elevation can be used with a topographic map to help ascertain your location and field landmarks.

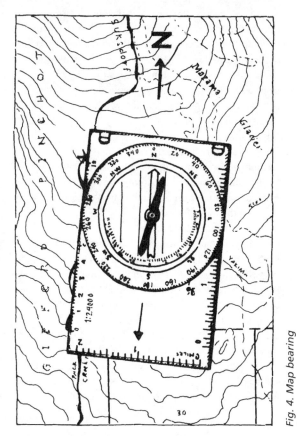

Fig. 4. Map bearing

An altimeter is basically a barometer that changes with both elevation changes and weather changes. It should be calibrated at places of known elevation such as the trailhead, campsite, or summit. If the weather changes overnight, you may need to recalibrate your altimeter in the morning. When the atmospheric pressure increases, the altimeter can show a false decrease in elevation, and vice versa.

Global Positioning System

The global positioning system (GPS) is a relatively new technology that is beyond the scope of this book. This electronic unit locates position by gathering reference data from both navigational satellites and way points that are programmed by the user.

You need a map and programmed way points or your GPS unit will be useless. Remember, electronic units can fail from water or cold exposure or dead batteries or being crushed. Also, deep canyons or other geologic and meteorologic phenomena can block access to satellites and render the unit useless. You must carry and know how to use a map, an altimeter, and a compass.

Shelter

Like procuring water, shelter is a high priority. In general, find shelter in a dry protected area such as a stand of heavy timber, a cave, or a cliff base. If in the mountains, try to get below timberline to minimize exposure. If in the desert, try to find shade.

There are numerous methods and techniques for shelters. A tent is perhaps the best shelter. A bivouac sack is a lightweight portable shelter. Common survival shelters include the following:

1. Rolled in a tarp, you can withstand a night in mild weather.
2. Using trees and a tarp, you can fashion a simple shelter (fig. 5). String cord between trees. Lay your tarp over

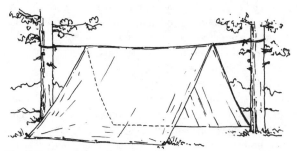

Fig. 5. Tree and tarp shelter

the rope and weight down the edges. Use downed limbs and foliage to make a sleeping platform. This will help insulate you from the ground.

3. If downed materials are plentiful, you can fashion a lean-to from logs and tree bows (fig. 6). Tie a rope or stick between two trees. Gently stack sticks against the crossbar.

4. Use a tree well to create a shelter using a tarp or downed bows stacked along the lower branches (fig. 7). This also works in the snow.

5. In the mountains, the simplest shelter is a snowtrench (fig. 8). Dig a 7-foot by 3-foot rectangular trench about 1 foot deep. Stack 2-foot by 2-foot snow blocks in A-frame fashion. Leave an opening to crawl in that you can block with a pack.

6. A snowcave is a larger, more complex shelter for two people or for multiple nights (fig. 9). Dig a 3-foot by 3-foot hole in a snowbank. Hollow out the inside enough for one or two people. Try to make the sleeping platform higher than the door. Once constructed, poke a hole or

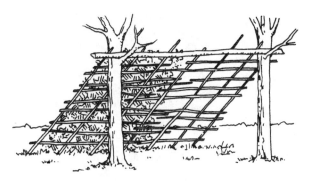

Fig. 6. Log and tree lean-to

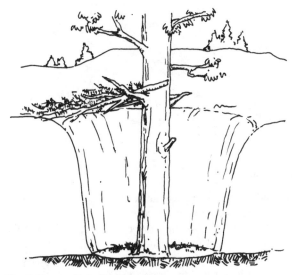

Fig. 7. Tree-well shelter in snow

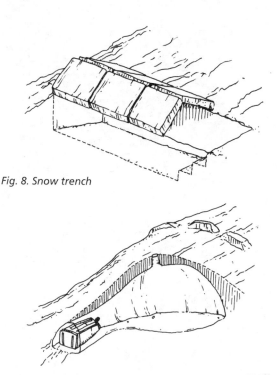

Fig. 8. Snow trench

Fig. 9. Snow cave

two in the roof for ventilation and use your pack to block the door to keep cold air out.

7. In the desert, the simplest shelter is a sand pit, or shade trench (fig. 10). Dig a 7-foot by 3-foot trench about 2 feet deep. Cover with a tarp, weighed down by sand at the edges. Carefully crawl in.

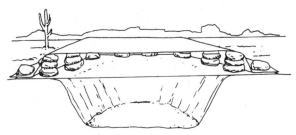

Fig. 10. Shade trench

Fire

Fire is a lower priority for survival in the wilderness than are water and shelter. It is useful for warmth, cooking, boiling water, and signaling. However, it can be labor intensive and difficult to build. Use the following steps:

1. Gather dry wood: only downed wood no thicker than your arm. Gather small, dry twigs and leaves for kindling and tinder.
2. Make a low-impact fire pit by clearing away brush, or use a dry river bed. Find a sheltered area out of wind and rain.
3. Place paper and a small candle or fire starter in the fire area. First-aid gauze soaked with petroleum jelly-based lip balm or sunscreen may work for fire starter.
4. Stack tinder (material that, if dry enough, should start from a spark).
5. Ignite fire starter or tinder using matches or lighter, shielding from wind and rain if necessary. Without matches, you can create a spark using flint and a steel knife blade. Often flints are located on match containers or come with your fire starter. Using a bow and drill to

twist a stick against a piece of wood is time consuming and difficult, but possible. With much luck, it may be possible to light tinder or fire starter with a magnifying glass that may be on your compass.

6. Once lit, slowly stack on more tinder and then kindling.
7. Blow on fire as needed.
8. Once you are finished, douse ashes with water or dirt. Scatter cold, wet ashes and remove your fire ring or pit.

Human Waste

Human waste is an important issue in survival, especially with regard to hygiene. There are several accepted methods for disposing of human waste. Deposit waste at least 300 feet from water sources. Either dig an 8-inch hole and bury waste, or smear it over dirt and rocks where sun and air can decompose it. Bury, burn, or carry out toilet paper. Use leaves if needed instead of toilet paper, but make sure they are not poison oak, ivy, or sumac! Above all, wash your hands afterward to prevent transmission of germs.

Procuring Food

Food is a low priority for survival. Fishing or hunting without proper tackle or equipment is very difficult. Snares and traps can be constructed from downed sticks and logs and rope or wire, if available. Fish can be caught from hooks and line if you have them, using worms or grubs for bait. Edible plants are plentiful, but you must know how to identify them. Don't eat plants if you don't know what they are. A common option in survival situations is eating insects, grubs, and worms.

Special Climates

There are numerous special climates that change priorities and techniques. These are beyond the scope of this book but are outlined briefly.

Deserts pose particular problems with heat and sun injury (see Other Medical Emergencies). Water procurement can be the number-one priority and can be accomplished using a solar still as outlined under Procuring Water. Seeking shade is also difficult due to lack of materials. A sand trench is described under Shelter.

Tropical and jungle environments pose problems with heat, as well as insect-borne diseases such as malaria. Cover all exposed skin using mosquito-proof clothing and headgear. Use mosquito nets for sleeping. Use insect repellent to avoid being bitten and inoculated.

Mountains pose problems with cold weather, lack of water, avalanches, shelters, acute mountain sickness, and lack of firewood. For the most part, these special situations have been incorporated into this text (for example, building a snowcave or snowtrench, procuring water by melting snow, and avoiding cold- and altitude-related illnesses). Specialized mountain rescue techniques such as crevasse or avalanche rescue are not included here.

Open ocean survival is complex and quite different from land survival. It is well beyond the scope of this book. The hazards are many and require further research by the reader. Fresh water can be acquired with a portable, handheld desalinator. If unavailable, a solar still similar to the one described for desert use can be constructed. Flotation is dependent on a life preserver, life raft, or boat. If nothing is available, survival floating and swimming techniques should be employed. Cold water is deadly, and a survival suit, if available, provides some protection. Hazardous marine life is abundant and includes predatory sharks, stinging jellyfish, and poisonous fish. Because there is little shelter available from weather, your boat is usually the best and only shelter at hand. Special signal devices may be on board, such as flares, flags, or an electronic emergency position-indicating radio beacon.

✦ Major Trauma ✦

Major trauma is something we hope never to encounter. However, when it occurs, it can be life threatening to the injured person as well as to partners attempting a rescue and first aid. Take a course in first aid. Many of these techniques should be employed only if you are properly trained.

General Evaluation

Approach all accidents in an orderly, stepwise fashion. Important: Do not move the injured person if there is risk of head or spine injury.

1. Avoid additional injury to the injured person, and avoid injury to rescuers.
2. Initiate primary survey. Evaluate airway, breathing, circulation, and disability. Initiate lifesaving measures such as CPR or bleeding control.
3. Initiate secondary survey. Complete a head-to-toe

evaluation for other injuries, including shock, wounds, fractures, dislocations, contusions, and hidden injuries.

4. Make a plan for continuing the trip, self-evacuation, or getting help, as outlined under General Survival Procedures and Evacuation.

Cardiopulmonary Resuscitation (CPR)
Signs and symptoms: No breathing and/or no pulse.
CPR Guidelines for those certified in CPR:
1. Make sure the scene is safe.
2. Do not move patient.
3. Wear gloves and use a CPR mask.
4. Check to see if victim is responsive.
5. Alert partners and call 911 on a cell phone.
6. Open airway using head tilt-chin lift and check breathing.
7. Give two rescue breaths if patient is not breathing.
8. Check pulse if trained.
9. Start chest compressions if patient is not breathing or if no pulse is found.
10. Give 30 compressions for every 2 breaths.
11. Apply an AED (defibrillator) if available.

Major Bleeding
Signs and symptoms: Obvious bleeding, light-headedness, dizziness, fainting.
Treatment:
1. Put on gloves.
2. Apply direct pressure with gauze or clothing.

3. Elevate affected arm or leg.
4. Consider pressure dressing if trained. Do not put on a tourniquet.
5. Consider pressure points if trained.

Head Injuries

Signs and symptoms: Unconsciousness; depression to skull; bleeding or clear fluid leaking from ears or nose; unequal pupil size or reactivity; nausea and vomiting; disorientation; drowsiness; severe headache; bruise behind ear or around eye.

Treatment:
1. Treat for coexisting neck injury.
2. Evacuate.
3. Repeat evaluations frequently.

Spine Injuries

Signs and symptoms: Head injury, neck pain, bad fall, or obvious neck injury. This can be a minor injury turned disastrous if not handled correctly.

Treatment:
1. Don't move patient.
2. Immobilize patient using full spine precautions if trained; summon help if not trained.

Shock

Signs and symptoms: Weakness, light-headedness, cold and clammy skin, weak pulse, rapid breathing, confusion, and disorientation.

Treatment:
1. Lay the person down or make the person as comfortable as possible.

2. Look for and treat the underlying cause: bleeding, low or high core temperature, dehydration, head or spine injury, infections, acute mountain sickness, or other problems.

+ *Other Medical Emergencies* +

Wound Care
Signs and symptoms: Obvious wounds with pain, bleeding, redness.
Treatment: Purify plenty of water. Put on gloves. Irrigate wound with plenty of water using syringe to dislodge deep particles. Clean with antibacterial cleanser. Cover with antibiotic ointment. Dress with standard bandage, butterfly bandage, or gauze. Use a gauze roll, triangle bandage, or clean shirt to cover entire wound and bandage. Check wound often, watching for redness, pus, heat, swelling, or worsening pain. Make sure fingers and toes are warm and have normal color, temperature, and sensation, i.e., that nerves and blood vessels are not being pinched. Clean wound and change dressing daily.

Sprains and Strains
Signs and symptoms: Pain, swelling, redness, and discomfort immediately following a fall or twisting injury.
Treatment: Have the injured person rest for a few minutes. Inspect injured area for lacerations or other wounds. Elevate the leg. Apply a compression wrap such as an elastic bandage. If possible, apply snow or soak in cool stream, but be careful not to cause frostbite or skin irritation. Try anti-

inflammatory medication. After a rest, you may need to splint the injury as a fracture, as described under Dislocations and Fractures and in Table 9.

Dislocations and Fractures

Signs and symptoms: See Sprains and Strains above. In addition, look for deformity, severe pain, bruising, and a grating sound with movement.

Treatment: Follow guidelines for sprains and strains. Splint fracture or dislocation as in Table 9. Use clothing or sleeping pad for padding. Splint the injured area using internal frame backpack stays, sticks, poles, clothing, ice axes, or a malleable splint. Secure the splint with climbing webbing, rope, string, first-aid tape, clothing, elastic wrap, or triangle bandage. Check wound often, watching for redness, pus, heat, swelling, or worsening pain. Make sure fingers and toes are warm and have normal color, temperature, and sensation, ie., that nerves and blood vessels are not being pinched.

Table 9: Splints

Splint	Use
Sling and swath (fig. 11)	Collarbone, shoulder, arm
Forearm splint (fig. 12)	Forearm, wrist, hand
Buddy tape	Finger, toe
Long leg splint (fig. 13)	Leg, knee
Boot	Ankle, foot

Hypothermia

Signs and symptoms: Feeling cold, shivering, stiffness, poor coordination, fatigue, poor judgment, confusion, dizziness, slow speech, nausea.

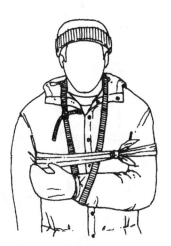

Fig. 11. Sling and swath splint

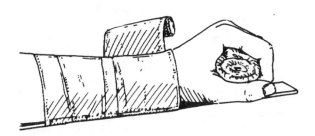

Fig. 12. Forearm splint

41

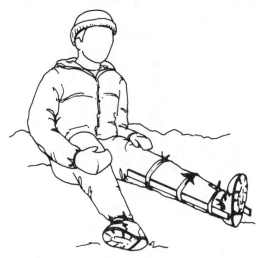

Fig. 13. Long leg splint

Treatment: Avoid cold and wet weather. Put on good-quality clothing and wear in layers, especially a hat, neck gaiter, gloves, and goggles. Change into dry clothing, especially socks. Find or build shelter, such as a tent, snowcave, or tree shelter. Get in sleeping bag or tent if available. Eat a snack and drink fluids, preferably a sport drink. Increase activity level to generate internal heat. Try chemical hot packs if available. Build a fire if possible.

Frostbite

Signs and symptoms: Cool, pale skin that is white or red. Site may be painful or numb and swollen. Blisters appear in advanced cases.

Treatment: Warm rapidly by placing in 40°C (104°F) water, if trained. Don't place near fire. Don't let the body part refreeze after thawing; it is usually better to evacuate with a frozen arm or leg than to have it refreeze. Anti-inflammatory medication will reduce pain and swelling. Pad arm or leg and splint as described under Dislocations and Fractures and in Table 9.

Acute Mountain Sickness
Signs and symptoms: Minor altitude illness includes headache, fatigue, weakness, dizziness, cough, nausea, shortness of breath, decreased appetite, and difficulty sleeping. Major symptoms include disorientation, poor coordination, severe breathing problems, vomiting, and severe headache. Life-threatening high-altitude pulmonary edema is marked by severe breathing problems, bluish skin, and loud cough with pink sputum. Life-threatening high-altitude cerebral edema is denoted by nausea and vomiting, difficulty thinking and speaking, dizziness and incoordination, and severe headache.
Treatment: Initially for minor symptoms, stop and rest. Drink fluids and eat some food. With any major symptoms or persistent minor symptoms, hike down to lower altitude immediately. Consider using anti-inflammatory medications. If you have prescription medications for acute mountain sickness, consider using them if you have been instructed how to do so.

Snowblindness
Signs and symptoms: Red, bloodshot, painful, light-sensitive, watery eyes. May be swollen.
Treatment: Wear sunglasses or goggles (fig. 14). Try anti-inflammatory medication. Improvise sunglasses by sticking

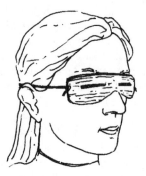

Fig. 14. Improvised goggles

together two strips of duct tape, cutting two slits for eye holes, and then tying around head with cord.

Heat Exhaustion

Signs and symptoms: Nausea, vomiting, dry skin, thirst, sweating, cramps, dizziness.

Treatment: Avoid midday heat. Drink fluids, preferably with electrolyte solution or sport drink. Wear light-colored, long-sleeved, long-legged clothes. Rest in the shade.

Heat Stroke

Signs and symptoms: See Heat Exhaustion. In addition, watch for shock, high temperature (over 40°C or 104°F), and mental status changes, such as slurred speech and confusion.

Treatment: Follow heat exhaustion guidelines. Also, begin cooling with water, such as misting skin, applying wet towels, and fanning.

Sunburn

Signs and symptoms: Red and painful skin.

Treatment: Wear sunscreen to prevent further injury. Apply liberally and often. Cover up using sun hat, long-sleeved shirt, long pants, and a bandana. Use aloe lotion. Anti-inflammatory medication may help.

Dehydration

Signs and symptoms: Headache, dizziness, fatigue, nausea, vomiting, and cramps.

Treatment: Drink fluids, preferably an electrolyte solution such as a sport drink.

Snake Bite

Signs and symptoms: Pain, redness, swelling, and bruising at site. Watch for dizziness, nausea and vomiting, fever and chills, and blurry vision.

Treatment: Clean as described under Wound Care. Apply a compression wrap if properly trained. Immobilize limb using a splint as described under Dislocations and Fractures and in Table 9.

Ticks

Signs and symptoms: Pain, redness, swelling, and achiness locally. Guard for dizziness, nausea, chills, and headache.

Treatment: Remove tick by using forceps. Grasp tick close to skin, and pull gently so as not to leave head in the wound. Clean as described under Wound Care.

Cardiopulmonary resuscitation courses are offered by the American Red Cross and at most community colleges.

Mountaineering is a general course on mountain skills, including mountain survival, such as snowtrench and snow-cave construction. Check with your local mountaineering club or outdoor store.

Mountaineering-oriented first aid (MOFA) provides mountain travelers with first-aid skills.

Wilderness first aid (WFA) is a course for basic first aid.

Wilderness first responder (WFR) is a longer, more detailed course designed for wilderness professionals.

Wilderness survival courses are plentiful around the country, ranging from one-day to week-long courses.

✦ Books to Read ✦

Angier, Brandford. *How to Stay Alive in the Woods.* New York: Fireside, 1998.

Backer, Howard, et al. *Wilderness First Aid: Emergency Care for Remote Locations.* Sudbury, MA: Jones and Bartlett, 1998.

Brown, Tom, Jr. *Tom Brown's Field Guide to Wilderness Survival.* New York: Berkley, 1989.

Craighead and Craighead. *How to Survive on Land and Sea.* 4th ed. Washington, DC: Naval Institute Press, 1984.

Darvill, Fred. *Mountaineering Medicine: A Wilderness Medical Guide.* 14th ed. Berkeley: Wilderness Press, 2000.

Davenport, Greg. *Wilderness Survival.* Mechanicsburg, PA: Stackpole Books, 1998.

Forgey, William. *Wilderness Medicine: Beyond First Aid.* 5th ed. Merrillville, IN: ICS Books, 2000.

Lentz, Macdonald, and Carline. *Mountaineering First Aid.* 5th ed. Seattle: The Mountaineers Books, 2004.

Swedo, Suzanne. *Wilderness Survival.* Helena, MT: Falcon, 1998.

Weiss, Eric A. *A Comprehensive Guide to Wilderness and Travel Medicine.* 2nd ed. Oakland, CA: Adventure Medical Kits, 1997.

Wilkerson, James A., M.D. ed. *Medicine for Mountaineering and Other Wilderness Activities.* 6th ed. Seattle: The Mountaineers Books, 2010.

Wiseman, John. *The SAS Survival Handbook.* London: HarperCollins, 1999.

Founded in 1906, The Mountaineers is a Seattle-based non-profit outdoor activity and conservation club, whose mission is "to explore, study, preserve, and enjoy the natural beauty of the outdoors...." The club sponsors many classes and year-round outdoor activities in the Pacific Northwest, and supports environmental causes by sponsoring legislation and presenting educational programs. The Mountaineers Books supports the club's mission by publishing travel and natural history guides, instructional texts, and works on conservation and history. For information, call or write The Mountaineers, Club Headquarters, 7700 Sand Point Way NE, Seattle, Washington, 98115; (206) 521-6001.

Send or call for our catalog of more than 500 outdoor titles:

The Mountaineers Books
1001 SW Klickitat Way, Suite 201
Seattle, WA 98134
800-553-4453
mbooks@mountaineersbooks.org
www.mountaineersbooks.org

The Mountaineers Books is proud to be a corporate sponsor of Leave No Trace, whose mission is to promote and inspire responsible outdoor recreation through education, research, and partnerships. The Leave No Trace program is focused specifically on human-powered (nonmotorized) recreation.

Leave No Trace strives to educate visitors about the nature of their recreational impacts, as well as offer techniques to prevent and minimize such impacts. Leave No Trace is best understood as an educational and ethical program, not as a set of rules and regulations.

For more information, visit *www.LNT.org,* or call 800-332-4100.

ISBN 978-0-89886-768-8

50350

32228

$ 2.18 $ 3.49⁹⁸

9 780898 867688